© 2022 Daina Mason

My Life With MND
Second Edition

ISBN: 9781739404420
Published by Experiments in Fiction
www.experimentsinfiction.com

Daina Mason

MY LIFE WITH MND

From diagnosis to daily life with Motor Neurone Disease

MY LIFE WITH MND

DAINA MASON

From diagnosis to daily life with Motor Neurone Disease

FOR MY HUSBAND BILLY, WITH THANKS FOR ALL OF YOUR LOVE AND DEVOTION

— DAINA MASON

About This Book

This book was written by Daina using eye-gaze technology, through which a camera picks up the motion of her eyebrows, which she uses to spell and select the correct words on her communication device. This is a slow and painstaking process, and as such serves as testament to her remarkable strength of character, fighting spirit, and positivity. It is this spirit which you will find throughout her story.

Note on the Second Edition

Since first publishing in December 2022, Daina's book has become an Amazon Bestseller, and helped healthcare workers determine future care plans for patients with MND. The book has also helped raise awareness of the condition, and raised money for vital MND research.

Daina has become famous on Radio Cumbria as 'MND Di' thanks to her tireless efforts to promote the book, and help others living with MND.

— *Ingrid Wilson, Publisher*

Contents

Chapter 1

From Early Symptoms to Diagnosis

The 29th of July 2014 started like any other day. Little did I know what was to come. My mum was in hospital after a bad fall, we'd had our tea, and as I had to pick up some clothes for my mum I set off, but got no further than the front door. I stepped out of the door and the next thing I knew I was on the ground: my leg just gave way underneath me. The funny thing was, I didn't feel any pain. I shouted for Billy, my husband. When he came out, he said, "what do you want me to do?"

"Get help would be nice!" I replied. He phoned for an ambulance. Of course, it came with full 'blues and twos.' The paramedics had a look at my ankle and said, "Is it always like that?" It didn't look bad, apart from a bulge at the front, so I told them "No." I was then put on a stretcher and loaded into the ambulance. Once inside, they tried to administer pain relief, although I still wasn't really feeling much in the way of pain. They couldn't find a vein in any case, so they gave me aspirin and gas and air until we got to A&E. By the time we arrived at A&E, I was shaking uncontrollably. The doctor said, "We can't x-ray you like that!" and gave me a shot of morphine, which did the trick. When they did the x-ray, they found my ankle was broken in three places, and also dislocated. I had evidently made a good job of it! The doctor then came back and said they were taking me to 'resus': that gave me a bit of a scare. I thought, "Am

I having a heart attack?" but it turned out that in order to reset the ankle, they had to put me under (almost, but not all the way) for whatever reason. They did tell me why, but I can't remember. The doctor said I wouldn't remember the conversation at all, so I think I did quite well remembering that much! After that, I was taken up to a ward. By this time, it was 9pm. I never did get to see my mum that day. The next morning, it was 'nil-by-mouth,' as the plan was to operate on my ankle in order to put the bones right. At 4pm, the nurse came with tea and toast, and said I could eat as I wouldn't be getting surgery that day. The next morning was the same again, 'nil-by-mouth.' That's one way to diet! This time, I went to theatre in the middle of visiting hours (about 2:30pm). When I came round after surgery, I was in plaster up to the knee, and I had several pins and a plate in my leg, which was now a bit sore. I spent a while in hospital until they were sure I could use the crutches, which I could in the hospital with its nice, even floors. The minute I got out of the car at home, I wasn't quite as confident, as the pavement wasn't so level. A few weeks later, my leg didn't feel right, so I went back to the hospital. They took the plaster off and x-rayed my leg again. They said everything was fine and put it back in plaster. After eight weeks, I went back for day surgery to get three of the pins taken out, and my leg was back in plaster for another eight weeks. By the time I was out of plaster, it was the end of November. My mum had passed away at the end of September, so it had not been a good year for me.

The first time I drove the car after breaking my ankle was Christmas day. I was very nervous, but it was not bad, so I felt things were getting back to normal. The stiffness in my ankle was still there, however, and it was sore at the end of the day. Something just didn't feel right. When I went to the doctor, he said everything was fine, so I thought, "OK, it's just me." Then my ankle started swelling by the end of the day, and it was really sore, so I took another trip to the doctor. Again, I was told there was nothing wrong with it, and so the situation continued for over two years. I even asked one doctor if I could be allergic to the plate that was in there, and she actually said, "Don't be stupid, there's nothing in there to be allergic to!" My ankle began to look like an elephant's leg. Eventually I saw a doctor who said, "You need that plate out!" which was a 'hallelujah moment.' The doctor I saw at the hospital was not very nice. He said, "What do you want me to do about it?" so I said, "Take it out!" To that, he said, "I suppose we'll have to do what you want." So, three years after breaking my ankle, I got the plate taken out.

As soon as the plate had been removed, the swelling in my ankle stopped. "Great!" I thought, "I can at last get back to normal." But the problems weren't over. My leg continued to be sore, and I started getting twitching in my legs and arms. At the time, I didn't give much thought to the twitching. It was only later I found out it was a symptom of MND. Once more, it was back to the doctors with - guess what? The same response: "There's nothing wrong." I persisted until I saw a doctor who took time to listen to me and think about my symptoms. She decided to test the reflex in my knee. Instead of my leg jumping when she tapped my knee, it made my whole leg shake. She said, "Let me think about it: there are two ways to go with this," then 20 minutes later she apologised for keeping me so long. I said, "Don't apologise, I'm just glad you're listening." She sent me for some tests. One was an MRI scan; another was to test how far signals travelled in my limbs. This test entailed strapping what I think were receivers on my wrists and ankles, then sticking probes into my arms and legs, and passing a small current in to see how long it took to get to the receiver. I must admit, when I saw the probe, I thought, "Oh no, this is going to hurt!" but I didn't feel a thing. These are the two tests I can remember. There were a few other bits, but they were mainly questions about different things. Then it was a waiting game for the results. I remember when I went for them, I thought at least I'd know what I was dealing with. When I was told they were inconclusive, and they would re-peat the tests in three months, I broke down and sobbed my heart out. When I managed to calm down, the consul-tant said, "Do you want a second opinion?" I said "yes." I got an appointment at the RVI in Newcastle, where I had to go through all the tests again. As a result of these tests, I ended up being diagnosed with MND on 30th July 2018, exactly four years and a day after I had broken my ankle.

Chapter 2

Adapting to Life with MND

Following on from my diagnosis, I was sent to the incontinence clinic, where I had to keep a diary of intake and out-take of my fluids. They supplied me with incontinence pads. Eventually I was referred to urology for Botox in the bladder but to get that, I needed to have more tests to see if I was suitable. These involved filling my bladder with water until it was full, then measuring how much came out. This was not the best of experiences! Then I went for the Botox which was "fun:" this time it was a camera in the bladder and a needle, and something to get hold of a bit of the wall of the bladder to inject the Botox into. The Botox was supposed to last 12 weeks until you needed to do it again. Mine lasted 5-6 weeks before I needed to go urgently and often again, so that was abandoned. Following on from this, in discussion with my consultant, we decided a catheter was the best way to go.

Meanwhile, my mobility was getting worse, so in February 2020 I got a hospital bed for my home and started sleeping downstairs. By the end of May, I started getting carers, and this worked well. I got the same two carers in the morning to get me up and showered, dressed and fed, then at night to put me to bed. I got on well with them. Then, at the end of September, the care company decided to change things, and bearing in mind this was in the middle of the pandemic, I started getting different carers. At first, it was a few different ones, which wasn't ideal, but not too bad to start with. In November, I ended up in hospital with a urine infection. The paramedics came just before 9pm and, as I was shaking a lot, they took me to A&E, where the doctor changed the catheter and tested my urine, then hooked me up to an antibiotic drip. I've got to say, it was quite entertaining a Saturday night in A&E, listening to the drunks with their excuses, "it wasn't me, honest, officer!" At 3am, I was moved onto a ward. At breakfast, they got me a coffee and toast and left me with it. Because my arms were now not very mobile, I didn't dare attempt the coffee and only managed a bite of toast, so when they came to take the cup and plate away they just said, "you finished," and took them away.

Moments later, there was a commotion in the ward opposite: a man was shouting, and the nurses were trying to calm him down. The next thing I knew, he came running through to the ward I was in and ripped something off the wall and was swinging it around at the nurses! Then a male nurse managed to get hold of him and get him back to his ward, but you could still hear him shouting. Then the police arrived and tried to calm him down. I don't know what happened next, but they pepper sprayed him and took him away. It was a long day! I think someone brought me a sandwich for lunch. I told them I couldn't manage to eat it myself as I couldn't get my arms up to my mouth, so they got someone to feed me. Just as the evening meal was about to come out, they came to move me to another ward. When I got my food again, I had to tell them I needed help. Then the drinks came, and I told the lady I couldn't manage on my own, so she tried a cup with a feeding lid. That was no good either, so she tried a straw through a hole on the top, and I could just about manage like that. Next was medication time: they had a copy of my medication, but the trouble was, one of them said 300g, but I was being built up to that dose, and I was only on 200g at the time. When the nurse brought 300, I explained this, and she shouted up the ward to the nurse giving them out, "she doesn't want these, she wants 200," then she went back and got the smaller dose, brought them back and dumped them on the trolley. This meant I had to buzz for someone to give me them. The worst thing was, of all the beds they could have given me, mine had no hand control, so every time I needed to sit up or lie down I had to buzz for someone to help me.

I settled down for the night. After what seemed like only a couple of hours, I was woken by the noise of someone having trouble breathing in another room: he was coughing and spluttering. My bed was at the entrance to the room, and there was no door. The entrance was opposite the room where the drugs were kept, and every time someone went in and out, the door would bang. They went in and out of that room a lot! I was also getting turned every couple of hours to stop me from getting bed sores, so I didn't get much sleep that night. The next morning, which was Monday, someone actually gave me a wash: my first since Saturday. Then it was time for breakfast. I had to ask for help again. A student nurse came, and after that, whenever she was on duty, she looked after me. The physio and a trainee physio came to see me. He said, "what happened to your hair? It's sticking up!" so I said, "like Bambam out of The Flintstones!" I told him it hadn't been brushed since I was brought to hospital, so the trainee found a comb and did it for me. Later, my speech therapist came to see me, as she'd seen my name on the admissions list.

She asked how I was doing, so I told her that I had to keep telling the staff I needed help. She wrote 'total assistance' on my name board, and after a chat, she left. Later that day, I watched some of the care assistants: you could see one or two of them take a look at the board and move on. You could almost hear them think, "I'll leave her for someone else." Later on, when the shifts were changing, I could hear the staff discuss who was doing extra shifts. I think they had all been working a lot. I heard one say she couldn't physically do any more shifts. The doctor came round and said all was looking good, and I could probably go home the next day. When it came to the drugs round, the nurse gave me the wrong dose of one of my tablets. It was one short, which was not going to hurt me, so I just thought, "it doesn't matter, I'm going home tomorrow," but the more I thought about it, the more I thought someone should know, in case a patient got ill because they'd been given the wrong medication. So, when the carer came to turn me, I told him. He said, "do you want me to report her?" I said, "no, as long as you know about it, I think she has enough going on as it is." Then I told him I was checking out of the Hotel Transylvania. He laughed and asked how many stars was I giving them? I said, "only two: it would have been less, but you had looked after me."

The next morning, I needed the toilet, so I buzzed for someone. A carer came, and I told her I needed the toilet. She said, "I'll bring a bed pan." I told her I couldn't sit on my own, and she said, "how we gonna get you there?" so I told her to bring a commode. Luckily, the trainee nurse came at that point and sorted it. With the help of two of them, they managed to get me on the commode and to the toilet and back to bed. Much later, the physios turned up. They wanted to know who I had at home and how I was going to cope. They wanted to see if I could transfer safely before I was allowed home. The first bit of equipment they brought was no good. I was quite a bit weaker after lying in bed for three days. Then they brought a return. I said, "I've got one of those at home, we had nicknamed it a sack barrow because that's what it looks like." With that, they got me out of the bed and into the chair. They were happy with that, so I was dressed ready for home and had to quickly ring Billy and tell him, "that sack barrow you said we would never use when the OT brought it? You better get it out of the garage as it's now an essential bit of kit that has to be in place for me to come home, and hopefully it wouldn't be long until I was there." We never disagreed with the OT when she said we should get something in place for when we needed it. Eventually, the hospital transport turned up. The trouble was, nobody had told them I couldn't walk into the ambulance, and the one they could push me into on the chair had been sent on another job, so I had to wait for that to get back. By the time I got home it was around 7pm.

The previous July, I'd had a catheter fitted. My consultant said it would be more comfortable for me to have a super-pubic one fitted, and that he would write to the urologist in Carlisle to arrange that for me. In August 2020, we had a break in covid restrictions, and, as travel was allowed again, we had a break to Oban in Scotland. My daughter had found a lodge on a caravan park belonging to MND Scotland that was fully equipped for me. So, we had that lodge with my daughter's family, and my son and his family got a lodge next to ours. My husband's brother and his wife came too. We had a fantastic holiday.

Back to the situation with carers: between October 2020 and the end of January, when the advice was not to mix with other households again, we had another 26 carers, which made 28 with the first two we had had. We kept saying, "this isn't right," but all we got from the company was, "we're following guidelines." Talking about guidelines, when the covid immunisation was being rolled out, it was by age and vulnerability. I never heard anything from my GP surgery, even though my MND team were saying I should get it sooner than by my age. I waited patiently, and eventually my husband was offered his first, as he's 11 months older than me. I was furious, so I rang the surgery and said, "can I ask where on the list am I?" The receptionist answered, "you're not due yet," so I said, "did they realise I had MND?" to which she replied, "I'm sure whoever decides these things will have looked at that." I told her they had made a mistake and I would speak to Mr Van-Tam, and they would be named and shamed, and then I put the phone down. I didn't do it, but it made me feel better.

Chapter 3

Continuous Care

Billy researched about NHS continuous care and applied for it. It's normally really hard to get, but for once, covid did us a favour: as we weren't allowed to attend meetings, the decision was made on the recommendation of the people who knew what they were talking about. I think the social worker had a lot to do with it, but we got it, and were given our own budget for carers. Not that it was easy to get the carers either, but at least there's a charity that takes care of payroll and any other admin, so we didn't have to grapple with all of that.

Last summer, my skin started getting itchy. I put it down to the heat, as it was a good summer, and I am stuck in my chair all day. My back was the worst. My daughter-in-law said, "try a dog cooling mat on your back." I borrowed one off her, and it worked to cool my back, so I made Billy get two.

In August 2021, we got the lodge in Oban again. We had a great holiday: I would recommend it to anyone with disabilities who likes to be in a scenic location with things nearby to visit. We even got the ferry to the Isle of Mull. Once again, we were lucky with the weather. My condition was getting worse, slowly but surely. I got visited by the district nurses regularly, and they were on the other end of the phone if we needed them. I finally heard from the hospital about the super-pubic catheter about 18 months after my consultant referred me for it. Billy took me to the hospital, which is an hour's drive away from where we live. I was told to be there for 12. We arrived a bit early and were told they were waiting for me. Once they did the paperwork and checked my blood pressure and things were OK, they took me to theatre to begin. The doctor said, "I'll just give you a local anaesthetic, and we'll begin." He wasn't joking: he had no sooner given me the local anaesthetic than he began. I felt everything. Luckily, it didn't take long.

The tube that went from the catheter to the bag must have been 5-6ft long, so the nurse that was discharging me said, "you don't want everyone seeing that on the way home," and found a carrier bag to put it in. She coiled the tube up and put it in the bag with the catheter bag, and we set off home. Not far down the road, I kept feeling uncomfortable as if my bladder was filling up, so I wriggled around until it eased up, but it kept doing it until finally, a mile from home, I was in agony. I told Billy as he pulled over to have a look: it had bypassed, and I was soaking. The tube must have got kinked when it was put in the bag. He got me sorted, and as it was a Saturday and his day for a few hours break from looking after me, he rang Helen my daughter to come and stay with me until he got back. After a while, my bladder started filling up again. It went again and when Helen had a look, it was blocked with what looked like a clot of blood, so she rang an ambulance. Before they came, it dislodged and started flowing again, so she cancelled the ambulance. Billy got home and heard all about it, and Helen went home: end of drama. A couple of hours later, the ambulance turned up. We had to explain what had happened, and they had to make a full report out instead of being able to get on to the next job.

Chapter 4

Staying Positive

There have been some good things which happened since I became ill with MND. After my broken ankle was healed, I started going swimming to strengthen it. Billy dropped me off at the pool, I did an hour's swim, then I rang him to pick me up. I did this three times a week. It worked well until my leg was much weaker, and I forgot my mobile. I knew Billy was nearby at my son's garage, so I thought I would be able to walk round there. I hadn't got very far when it became too difficult. I thought I was going to fall, and even if I could manage to hobble, there was a busy main road to negotiate, and I didn't trust my legs to get me over it, so I stopped to rest by a unit that sold second hand furniture. The man who owned it (I think) came out and asked if I was OK, so I explained what had happened and asked if I could use his phone. Bless him, he gave me his mobile and even got me a chair to sit on while I waited! In true comedy style, I rang the garage, and Claire, my daughter-in-law answered and said Billy had gone to collect something for them, so she would come for me. While I was waiting for her, sat on a chair on the pavement, I saw Billy pass the road end on the way to the pool. Of course, he didn't look down the road where I was. I thought, "he'll come this way to get back to the garage." He didn't, so I watched as he passed again. Claire turned up, and I tried to see the man inside to say thank you, but didn't see him, so if he reads this: a big thanks!

After I was diagnosed, we attended the clinic to see the consultant at Penrith where the MND volunteers welcomed us and gave us a coffee and a biscuit, and the all-important chat. It turned out that Penrith hospice ran a day-care session once a week in the hospital, and they did a swimming trip to the Calvert trust pool once a month. I was able to join them on the swimming trip: the pool is fully equipped for disabled people, so I jumped at the chance, and the volunteers even helped me get dressed. Of course, covid put an end to that. We used to have a support group as well: we met every second month, but that stopped with covid and never started again. At least the walks that were organised by a lady whose husband died from MND restarted when restrictions were lifted. It's a chance to meet up with other people. I also got a monthly hand and foot massage, which also restarted when restrictions were lifted. Hospice at home provide this. Instead of the massage, I decided to have reflexology, which someone told me was good. I must admit I wasn't sure if it would work, but I was wrong. I swear the woman who did it had magic fingers! I would highly recommend it now, but she retired during covid, so I'm back to massage. The lady that does that is really nice too.

Just after Christmas 2021, I got a bad chest. I couldn't get rid of it, whatever I tried. The MND coordinator got me a nebuliser, which helped, but didn't get rid of it. I went through five lots of antibiotics, five courses of steroids and a chest x-ray, and I only got to see a doctor for the first time in three years (apart from my hospital visits) before the last course of antibiotics. At the end of May, it cleared up as quickly as it had started. I try to stay positive, but sometimes it just gets me when I think of what I'm reduced to. I can't even scratch an itch now. I used to do all sorts of crafts. In fact, at one time, I was spending a lot of money on craft supplies. Billy looked at the bank statement and said, "how much?" I found out it's a symptom of MND: as you lose control of your body, you try to compensate by having control over your spending, or even overcompensate by overspending.

Chapter 5

Mixed Emotions

In late August, we had our holiday again, this time we tried the MND lodge near St Andrews. It was very good: there was a pool to use, a shop and a bar that served food and had entertainment in the evening, so in that way it had more than the Oban site, but I did like the scenery better at Oban, although that's just my opinion. In September, I was having trouble with my catheter, which was a bit of an ongoing problem. The district nurse came and said, "we're going to try a different catheter," and she pulled the old one out, but when she tried to get the new one in, it wouldn't go in, so she rang a colleague who came with a smaller one. In the end, they got one in two sizes smaller than I'd had in previously. Within half an hour of them leaving it bypassed again, so back they came. They didn't want to change it in case it wouldn't go back in, and because of the chance of infection, so they left it in and fitted another by the normal way, then arranged for urology to see me the next day in emergency day care. So, for the rest of the evening, I had two catheters in, one strapped to each leg. I said to Billy, "it's like having twin exhausts fitted." The next morning, the doctor tried to put in the same size as I'd had to start with, but he had to settle for the size below, and he said, "we'll go up a size in eight weeks' time. Meanwhile, we'll put a camera in to see what's going on." Billy said, "can you do that now?" So he said, "in an ideal world, but we're not in an ideal world, so you'll get an appointment for that."

I used to joke with my mother about doing a tour of the hospital, but I reckon I've beaten her on that one. I was pretty healthy until I was 51, when I went for my first mammogram, where they found a lump in my right breast. I recovered from that after all the treatment and was discharged after five years only to go back the sixth year to find one in the left side. With treatment, recovered from that also, but I guess my luck ran out with MND.

Harder to talk about are the emotions you go through. They range right through from the top to the bottom. The day you get the diagnosis, you are in a state of shock and disbelief. Once you get over that bit, you think, "right, let's take a day at a time and enjoy what I can do for as long as possible." The first thing to go was my gardening. I kept it going for as long as I could. I would get down on my knees. I bought knee pads and crawled along the border of flowers, weeding until I got round the garden. Once I gave it up, Billy had to do it, which wasn't too bad, but I dread it when I see him with the secateurs in his hand. His idea of gardening is to hack everything down, never mind at what time of year it's supposed to be done! At least I still had my crafting I could do to keep me happy. I do get days when it hits me that I can no longer do something when I just hit rock bottom and sob my heart out, then I think "this isn't doing any good, I'm only hurting myself," so I pick myself up and get on with doing the things I can still manage. One of the hardest things is losing the ability to speak. It can be funny as well when people try to guess what you're saying and get it wrong. I try again, and it's like a game of charades. Sometimes I just get the giggles and can't get it out until I calm down again. The hardest time is when there are a few people, and they are all chatting, and I can't join in. By the time I type a comment out on my communication device, the conversation has changed topic I tried a couple of times and everyone just looked blank because it just sounded so random, so I don't try now. It can feel very isolating. I'm on the sidelines now, and I used to be in the thick of it. Poor Billy suffers the most, as once the carers have finished in the morning, he's the one to do everything until bedtime.

Sometimes he's up and down like a yo-yo, especially in the evening, as when I've been sat in my chair all day, I get stiff and need my arms stretched out as the pressure makes them go to sleep. He says I do it on purpose, but I don't, honest!

Chapter 6

My Current Situation

I have to say that without Billy it would be much worse. He's left with most of the work, and if you'd have told me he would be doing everything for me that he does now I'd have said, "no way," but he's stepped up to the plate, and then some. We get carers in the morning and at bedtime, and we would qualify for more, but you can't get carers that are good unless you go with a care company, and even they struggle to keep staff. You end up not knowing who or if anyone is coming, as we found out, and the good ones get sick of being messed around and leave. We have managed to get two carers and get family to try and fill the gaps, but they have jobs and families, and if one of my carers is off sick the other helps out when they can, but one's a student, so she fits in around her studies, and the other has family, and life happens. She's not well at the moment, so Billy gets a lot of the work. A lot of the help I need is with little things like getting drinks, or scratching an itch, or late afternoon my arms start needing moved because they go numb with being in the same position all day, so I manage to keep him busy. We keep joking, "who needs a gym when he's got me?" I'm hoping my carer will be back, as she's become a friend too, but it looks like it could be quite a while until she's fit to return, so we're having to look for someone else, which isn't easy given the stage I'm at. A lot depends on knowing what I need and understanding my nods and grunts when I'm not on my device.

I've just been to have my feeding peg fitted for when I can no longer eat and drink, as it will become more difficult to do that. Before I go into the details of what went wrong, I'll just say that all the staff were absolutely lovely. The problems happened because I'm totally dependent on others to do everything for me, and if my communication device has been moved, there's no way for me to tell anyone what I need. The fact that they were short-staffed didn't help either. I went into hospital on Friday afternoon, and stayed in my wheelchair while Billy set my device up on the trolley that goes over the bed, so we didn't get to try it with me in bed. When Billy had gone home, I had my dinner and then was put to bed. The communication problems started every time someone came to check my blood pressure or take blood. They moved my arm, which moved the clicker I use on my thumb. This works with my glasses: they have a dot on which is picked up by the camera on the device, which I move to the letter on the screen, and when I get to the one I want, I click with my thumb against the side of my hand. As I have very little movement, it has got to be set just right, so as I said, every time it was moved and not put back just right it was a big problem for me. The weekend wasn't too bad, apart from the fact that with each shift change, I had to go through the process of getting the new staff to understand my needs. On Saturday night, the window was left open all night. I think some of the patients and staff were too hot. Unfortunately, it set my chest off. To start with it was just a little cough, but it kept getting worse each day, so on Monday I told Billy to bring my Ventolin inhaler from home. I never thought of asking the nurses for one. By Tuesday morning, the doctors on their rounds said the cough was getting worse. I explained I'd told Billy to bring the inhaler in and one doctor said, "you don't have to wait for that, we can get one," so they did this, but they also sent me for a chest x-ray. Once I got the inhaler, my chest was OK. After midnight on Sunday, I was nil-by-mouth, and Monday morning I was taken for the procedure to get the peg fitted. By the time Billy came for visiting at two o clock, I was back on the ward. I was awake for the operation, and it only took ten minutes to fit.

More blood was taken. I said to the doctor, "I'm sure you're all vampires," so we called him Dracula, and the other one that kept coming for bloods got called Dr Blood. It ended up as the worst night ever. At six in the evening, I asked the nurse to move me as I was uncomfortable. She said she would be back in five minutes. It was busy, with buzzers going off all the time, so I guess she forgot about me. I got the woman in the bed opposite me to buzz, but I got the same response. Someone finally came at midnight to move me. It was fine for a while, but one of my arms was stuck half under me, so I tried getting the attention of someone to move it, but they were rushing around and didn't hear me. Then I got heartburn, and at around two am, I got pains in my chest that kept coming and going. Finally, just before six in the morning, someone came to check on me, and then it was all action. My hand and arm were swollen with being trapped, so they sorted that and got a machine to get my heart checked and sent for a doctor. After breakfast and a wash and my teeth cleaned (that was hit-and-miss: out of six mornings I got my teeth cleaned three times, and not once at night) they decided I was to be put in a chair for a while as the pressure sores on my bottom were starting to open up with lying in bed all the time. The trouble with that was the chair was so hard it felt worse. Just before visiting, the doctor came and said that I was OK, but I was to have an aspirin as they thought I'd had a little heart attack. Billy arrived as I was digesting that information. By this time, I was really uncomfortable in the chair, so they came to put me back in bed. We decided that if I couldn't get a nurse in future, I should message Billy, and he would phone the ward to tell them I needed help.

So, when the nurse decided I needed to get off the pressure sores on my bottom by laying me on my side with pillows to hold me in position, it was fine for the first half an hour, then I started getting sore where the peg was, so I typed in, "help nurse," as the woman who pressed her buzzer for me had been discharged earlier, so I just kept repeating help nurse for twenty minutes. I could hear them at the nurses' station, but no-one came over. I messaged Billy to help, but after ten minutes with no response from him, I thought, "Helen always hears her mobile," so I just sent, "help!" to her. Billy hadn't told her what the plan of action was, but I didn't know that. She told me later she got such a shock when she saw the message, but it worked because I could hear the nurse talking to her saying, "yes, I can see her, she's fine," and I'm lying there thinking, "I'm not." But once she came off the phone, she came to see me and I told her what the problem was, and she moved me. The next morning, at 7:40, my catheter bypassed. I managed to get hold of someone at 8:20 and told her I'd bypassed. To my amazement, she said, "we're all busy with breakfasts, you'll have to wait." So, wait I did, through breakfast and beyond. My device had got moved again, so when my consultant came to see me and tell me that they'd looked at everything and didn't think I'd had a heart attack, and it was probably angina, so they were trying to get me home, all I could do was nod. At last, just before lunch, they came to give me a bed bath and put dry sheets on. Once again, I could hear them on the phone discussing my transport. They were saying I needed a stretcher transport. I thought, "why, what's wrong with my wheelchair?" When Billy arrived at two for visiting, he asked why I wasn't going home in the wheelchair, and the ward manager said she'd asked if I had a wheelchair and had been told there wasn't one, so Billy told her it had been by my bed the whole time! We were waiting for the meds to come from the pharmacy, and we would be ready to go when the transport came, but they couldn't take Billy, so he said, "never mind, I'll get the bus and arrange for someone to be at the house." As it happened, the transport arrived ten minutes later. The meds hadn't arrived yet, so Billy said he would wait for them. Off we went. Billy came down to the ambulance with the wheelchair. On the way down, when we got in the lift, there was a policeman already in. I said, "I'm getting a police escort as well." Poor Billy: when the meds arrived, he had four full bags to carry, as they'd sent all the supplement drinks I had to take for the next month! He said his arms were shaking by the time he got to the bus.

That was the end of my stay in the all-inclusive five-star hotel known as the hospital, where not only did I get fed and watered, but they even gave me a free spa treatment called 'colonic irrigation.' I got that on the Sunday night before the peg was fitted, and, oh my days! I didn't know you could have so much stored in there. So at least I was home now, and I only had to get through Tuesday at the local hospital where they were going to put a new catheter in after the twin exhaust event. Of course, that didn't go well. Why would it? This is me, after all! We got to the hospital with ten minutes to spare, or so we thought. We went to the back entrance where all the disabled parking is, but it was busy with three cars already waiting to park, so we waited in the queue. By the time we were next, we were running late for my appointment, so Billy said, "I'll park at the door and get you up to reception, then I'll come back and move the van." He left the back doors open and the ramp down, so it would be obvious that a patient was being delivered.

But things are never straightforward for us! When

we got to the department, we were told to go to reception, and they said, "no, you're not here," and sent us to the other end of the atrium, where we explained that we'd been sent there, so at least the receptionist said, "I'll find out what's going on," so Billy said, "I'll have to move the van. I'll be straight back." When he got back, you could see the steam coming out of his ears: the jobsworth parking attendant had given him a ticket! When Billy queried it with him, he just said, "you're not an ambulance" and walked away. But the definition of 'ambulance' is 'a vehicle for the transportation of patients.' We should have ordered hospital transport and that wouldn't have happened. Meanwhile, the woman came back and told us we had been in the right place at first and sent us back there. They weren't ready for us, even though they should have been as we had an appointment, and they should have known what we were there for. Eventually, they found a room for us, then they had to find a portable hoist. The consultant turned up with the gas and air, as last time it took ages to organise that. After some time, they were ready to start, only the balloon that gets inflated in the bladder at the end of the catheter to stop it from coming out when it's not supposed to wouldn't deflate. He was pushing and pulling it, but it wasn't going anywhere, so he went and got a portable ultrasound scanner to see what was going on. By this time, we'd been in the hospital three hours. Billy didn't want another parking ticket, so he said he'd have to go and sort the parking display out. No sooner had he left to do that than I got a lot of pain, and the consultant said he'd managed to get the old catheter out and the new one in. My guess is that after trying for forty minutes he was sick, and when Billy left the room, he just yanked it out. He even apologised for my pain. A week and a half later, I'm still having problems, and the poor district nurses are left trying to sort me out.

*** ***

I'm now at the stage where I can't do much of anything. Thank goodness I've got my device. I keep my mind occupied with card games and reading books on the device. I can get emails and WhatsApp, and don't think about how long I have left. Last year while lying awake at night I was thinking, "how can I do something to raise funds for research?" I can't run marathons like my daughter: she also sells excess plants in the spring from a bench outside her home, and she's signed up for the Rob Burrows full marathon in Leeds next May, the day after I turn 70. I can't climb mountains, so I thought, "I know, I can have my head shaved!" By the morning, I had it all worked out: do it in the centre of town on the August Bank holiday while Carlisle had a food fair on to maximise crowds and get as much media involved as I could. I didn't know how badly my family would react! They said it was hard enough seeing me deteriorate without seeing me with no hair, but I was still up for it. In the end, I was persuaded to open a JustGiving page and let people have a vote to shave or not for a donation. I lost the vote: I still maintain it was rigged by them! We had a coffee and cake afternoon on the August Bank holiday instead, and any cake left over, Helen took around her neighbours. Everyone was really generous, and we made just over £1,500. I still think I should have shaved my head! My little grey cells went to work again, and I came up with the idea with a little help from my neighbour to write this account of my journey with MND. My niece publishes books, and she said she would publish my story, and use it to help raise awareness, and also raise funds for research, as without the research there will never be a cure for what is a very cruel disease.

Printed in Great Britain
by Amazon

31634574R00030